60 Tips for a Slimmer & Healthier You

Look Better, Feel Younger, Live Longer!

(Volume 1)

Legal Notice

This publication is not intended to be used as a source of Health & Fitness advice.
The purchaser or reader assumes responsibility for the use of these materials and information. Pete Lyons (DBA Get Fit Personal Training) assumes no responsibility whatsoever on behalf of the purchaser or reader.

Disclaimer

The information contained in this publication (e-book) is designed to help you make informed decisions about your health. It is not intended as a substitute for any treatment prescribed by your doctor. If you suspect that you have a medical problem, please seek competent medical care immediately.

Before you undertake a new health program or fitness regimen, you should consult with your health care professional, especially if you have not exercised before or for several years, are over age 35, and/or are overweight.

The purchaser or reader is responsible for the way this information is perceived and utilized and done so at your own risk. In no way is Pete Lyons (DBA Get Fit Personal Training) responsible for any injuries or health problems that may occur from the use of the advice contained in this material.

Copyright Notice

Introduction

Thank you for purchasing my book! You have taken a very important step in your life-to improve your health. If you read through my book thoroughly and put these tips into practice, I promise you will be feeling and looking significantly better. As you know, there is a TON of information available in various forms about health and fitness. I wanted to create a simple, straightforward and valuable resource for that you can put immediately into practice today. These tips are from what I have learned, personally practice and have taught in my nine years in the fitness industry coaching and training clients.

Our country is getting unhealthier each year. Health-related diseases such as diabetes, hypertension, cardiovascular disorders, and various cancers are at an all-time high. We must be aware of the effects that obesity and inactivity has on our bodies as well as the psychological effects on our self-esteem and confidence. Many of these diseases are preventable if we just make better nutrition choices and add some daily exercise. I believe that the best way to prevent these negative effects it is at your local supermarket where superfoods and amazing nutritious foods are sold. That together with daily exercise can have an astounding impact on how you look and feel without the use of pills and fads that are commonplace today.

Most people know that daily exercise and eating healthy are beneficial. Many have good intentions and decide to make some changes. However, the biggest problem is that it is usually short-lived. Our struggle lies in the challenge of keeping excess weight off and continuing a healthy nutrition plan long-term. It is a complex process that takes discipline and sacrifice initially, but once you establish a strong foundation you will be successful and able to live life to its fullest!

There are <u>four key ingredients</u> to a well-rounded healthy lifestyle: Cardiovascular exercise, strength training, healthy nutrition, and the right mindset. The tips on the following pages will involve all of these and provide you with valuable information you can put into practice right away.

I recommend that you start with one or two of the tips per week and don't try to change too much too soon. Establishing long-term healthy habits takes some time so don't stress over it. Realize that you will always be a "work in progress" as unexpected lifestyle changes and other things will inevitably come at you and force you to adapt. Some of these tips may already be part of your lifestyle-good for you! If so, use it as a reminder of how valuable it is and keep practicing them. Finally, never forget that *"Your Health Is Your Greatest Wealth".*

Now let's dive into those tips!

Yours in Good Health,

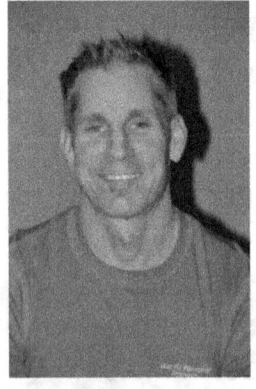

Pete Lyons
ACE Certified Personal Trainer
Owner, Get Fit Personal Training

Like my Facebook page:
www.facebook.com/getfitpt

Follow me on Instagram: Trainhard2day

Beachbody coach page:
www.beachbodycoach.com/getfitpt

Have questions or comments? Email me: Pete@getfit-wa.com

60 Tips for a Slimmer & Healthier You

Look Better, Feel Younger, Live Longer!

(Volume 1)

Tip 1- Move!

This may seem obvious but the average person sits an average of 12 hours per day, which is A LOT of sitting! Combine this sedentary habit with poor nutrition and a lot of health problems are the result. Some of these include heart disease, stroke, high blood pressure, and joint pain just to name a few. In addition, all that sitting shortens muscle fibers, decreases flexibility, decreases blood flow throughout the body, and causes lethargy, digestion problems and numerous other issues. The American Heart association recommends adults get 150 minutes of moderate aerobic exercise per week or 75 minutes of vigorous exercise (or a combination of both). Unfortunately, around 80 % of adults in the US do not meet this recommendation.

As little as 20 minutes per day of exercise can provide health benefits. The type of exercise should depend on each person's ability, lifestyle, and physical limitations. For a beginner exerciser, walking outdoors and adding small hills would be a good place to start. For more advanced exercisers, things such as jogging, sprints, HIIT, or swimming would be good options. Discuss your intentions with your healthcare provider and ask for recommendations.

Tip 2- Drink More Water

Approximately 70 percent of your body is made up of water. Even your bones are one-quarter water. The fact is that most people are chronically dehydrated because they just don't drink enough water. Unfortunately, our choices for drinks and quenching thirst have become soda, fruit juices, energy drinks and hundreds of other products that food companies market incessantly. These beverages contain massive amounts of sugar, artificial flavors, and other artificial ingredients that can become detrimental to our health.

Why do we need to drink water? Water goes beyond being a thirst quencher as it aids in healthy skin, building muscle, controlling calories, flushing toxins from the body, and improving digestion. Water also plays an important role in weight loss. Drinking a lot of water may sound counterintuitive for weight loss, but doing this flushes water out of the body that it may be retaining. You may notice body composition changes in the hips, thighs, ankles, and even around your belly. This is why when you lose weight, a percentage of the loss is from water.

My recommendation is to drink 1/2 of your bodyweight in ounces. (i.e.: If you weigh 150 lbs., your target should be around 75 ounces per day). To get on the right track, make it a habit to drink a large glass of water as soon as you wake as this will help to jump-start your metabolism, feed your organs, and hydrate you after a 7 or 8 hour fasting state.

Tip 3- Control Sugar Intake

Sugar is added to just about everything you eat these days. It is very important to control how much you consume daily. The troubling fact is that you don't even know you are consuming it because it is hidden in most foods. It is important to note that I am referring to "added sugar" which is added during the processing or preparation of foods and beverages. This is different from "natural sugar" that is naturally found in fruits (fructose), milk (lactose) and other dairy products. The USDA recommends that you consume no more than six teaspoons of added (refined) sugar for women and no more than nine teaspoons for men. Unfortunately, The USDA's most recent figures find that Americans consume, on average, about 32 teaspoons of added sugar every single day, yikes! Sugar has become an addiction much like a drug for millions of people in this country.

What dangers do we face eating too much sugar? First, sugary foods will increase your body's demand for insulin- a hormone that helps your body convert food into usable energy. If you are sedentary or not very active, this energy most likely won't be used and it will be stored as fat, especially around the belly. Further, when insulin levels are consistently high, your body's sensitivity to the hormone is reduced and glucose builds up in the blood- not what you want. In addition to obesity, excess sugar can lead to diabetes, heart disease, hypertension and other serious health issues and diseases.

The best advice I can give to you is to read food labels and swap out sugary foods and beverages with fresh fruits and vegetables as much as possible. Finally, use apps such as MyFitnessPal to keep track of sugar in your diet and review it weekly.

Tip 4- Hire a Coach

Notice how I said "coach" and not "trainer". Nowadays, there are literally thousands of fitness sites on the internet and apps giving you advice on exercises, nutrition, how to get rid of belly fat, and how many calories you should be eating etc. Anyone can use google to obtain information. What you need MORE than this stuff is someone to guide, support, and educate you on how to apply this information and put yourself in the right mental state. Maintaining healthy habits can be difficult to stick to long term, however having someone as a coach to motivate and hold you accountable is invaluable.

Some other reasons why hiring a coach would benefit you:

- Nutritional advice and recommendations
- Body composition assessments
- Proper exercise form and modifications (if needed)
- Support and Accountability
- Variety of exercises and equipment

Tip 5- Strength Train

Strength training (resistance or weight training) is absolutely critical for a well-rounded fitness plan. There are a lot of benefits associated with strength training. Some of these are an increase in muscle size, strength, weight loss and/or management, increased metabolic rate, injury prevention, better balance, decreased risk of heart and other diseases, increasing bone density, and most important feeling and looking better so you can enjoy life and not suffer from chronic pain or injuries!

The leaner (more muscular) your body becomes, the more efficient it will be at increasing your metabolism and burning calories. Women, you will not get "big and bulky" from lifting weights! This is a common misconception. Women need strength training just as much as men for all the benefits described above.

If you are losing weight and not strength training you are also losing hard-earned, valuable muscle, definitely what you don't want. Strength training is one of the most important components of fat loss since muscle burns more calories, even at rest. Think of your body as a machine and your muscle as your "engine". The more muscle you have, the more efficient your body will be at burning calories, losing body fat, or maintaining your lean physique. For every pound of muscle you gain, your body expends approximately 50 extra calories per day.

Strength training can be done using various equipment such as medicine balls, dumbbells, stability balls, TRX suspension trainer, and kettlebells just to name a few. Your own bodyweight can be the perfect tool for an effective and convenient workout.

My recommendation is to strength train at least 2-3 times per week performing exercises that work your whole body.

Tip 6- Try HIIT Training

One type of Resistance training that has become very popular is HIIT (High Intensity Interval Training). HIIT is a type of training that involves short bursts of exercise (usually 30-60 secs) followed by short rest. It used to be taught that massive amounts of long-duration walks on the treadmill was what was needed to burn fat and maintain weight. However, in recent years studies show that shorter and more intense bouts of exercise are a lot more effective at burning fat and getting lean. This type of exercise puts your type 2 (fast twitch) muscle fibers to work, requires you to use your whole body, and increases your heart rate quickly giving you results in much less time.

What are some examples? Forty-yard sprints, jump squats, hill or stair runs, burpee/treadmill jog combo. Be sure to mix up your exercises and routines to keep it fun and maximize your results.

Tip 7- Sleep

The late night shows may be funny, but they're not worth the strain on your body from inadequate quality sleep. 7-8 hours of sleep per night helps to lower stress, sharpens memory, keeps you disciplined and on track, and will potentially help you to live a longer life.

Studies published in the Journal of the American Medical Association show that sleep loss disrupts a series of complex metabolic and hormonal processes which can make weight loss far more difficult. Further, sleep deprived and tired individuals tend to eat more during the day and make poorer food choices. You also need adequate sleep to repair those muscles and aid in recovery. Set a bedtime and stick to it. Shut off all electronics including iPhones, laptops, and tablets at least one hour before bedtime so your brain can become "unstimulated" and you can fall asleep faster.

Tip 8- Eat More Protein

Consuming protein benefits your body in many ways. First, it is essential for building and maintaining muscle. It also aids in the repair and recovery post-workout.

Protein keeps you feeling fuller longer because it takes approximately 25% longer for your body to digest, which can help with cravings and aid weight loss. Eating enough protein signals your body to make, and retain muscle and other lean tissue. Many clients ask me how much they should consume daily. This depends on several factors- activity level, diet restrictions, goals, age, and other considerations.

Protein sources should be from lean meats, fish, legumes and dairy products. It is always best to discuss your requirements with your doctor or nutritionist.

Tip 9- Self Development

Self-development is about taking steps to better yourself, such as learning new skills or overcoming bad habits. Educating yourself so that you can succeed spiritually, financially and emotionally are super important and should be a part of your daily routine.

Find some topics that are of interest to you and purchase some books or audio recordings. I recommend that you dedicate at least 30 minutes a day to self-development. Put this time on your daily calendar so you are more likely to stick to it.

Do it....Your future self will thank you!

Tip 10- Control Portions

It is very important to make sure you are watching your food portions, especially if eating out. Most restaurant's servings are 2-3 times more than you need! This can sabotage your daily calorie intake and lead to weight gain. Believe me, restaurants are in business to make food taste good and make money, your waist size is not a priority! Here are some ways to control portions:

1. Use a smaller plate. This way, you are less likely to eat more than you need.
2. Include meals well balanced with protein, whole grains or complex carbs such as fresh vegetables.
3. When eating out, request a box before your food arrives and take ½ home.
4. Share an entrée with someone.
5. Eat small, more frequent meals throughout the day.

More info and portion charts are available at http://www.usda.gov

Tip 11- Eat Fat!

It is a common myth that eating fat will make you fat. However, this is not totally true. You need to be eating the right types of fat. Healthy fats are those labeled monounsaturated and polyunsaturated. Examples of healthy fats are avocados, olive oil, coconut oil, flaxseed, walnuts and other raw nuts. These types of fats are essential for the body and help to keep cholesterol levels in the safe range. Healthy fats also have been proven to reduce the risk of certain diseases such as high blood pressure and atherosclerosis, balance blood sugars and reduce inflammation in the body.

Another form of healthy fats are Omega-3's. These fats can be obtained from your food sources or through supplementation. Omega-3 is most abundant in cold water fish such as salmon, mackerel and sardines, Flaxseed (linseed) oil.

You can also buy Omega-3 oil to supplement your diet if needed. Some other benefits of eating these types of fat is that they make you feel fuller in a small portion. This can be very important if weight loss is your goal. Other studies have shown that people who follow a higher fat diet are more successful at losing body fat and maintaining a healthy weight.

Finally, always avoid any foods that contain large amounts of Trans fats, which have been proven to cause obesity, atherosclerosis, and many other diseases. Aim to include approximately 20 % of your daily calories from these healthy fat sources but it is always best to check with your doctor or nutritionist to find out what is appropriate for you.

Tip 12- Journal

Keeping a journal is a valuable tool to record things such as daily experiences, workout progress, nutritional tracking, or anything you could find useful for future reference. Putting things in writing has been proven to further clarify your thoughts and gives you the opportunity to work through ideas/thoughts that may otherwise exist as rolling tumbleweeds in your head.

In addition, journaling will help you stay more focused and organized since everything is in one place. When you put things in writing, you are twice as likely to follow through with them.

Many medical professionals and institutions promote the use of journals as a method to pacify the "monkey mind"-managing emotions and reducing stress and anxiety. Head out tomorrow and get yourself a journal…it could be the best $15 you spend this year!

Tip 13- Eat Breakfast

Numerous studies continue to show that people who eat breakfast every day have lower body fat percentages. When you sleep, your body goes into a fasting state so when you awake you need to eat to get your metabolism started. In addition, your metabolism is naturally more effective at burning calories in the morning.

Your menu should include some protein and fiber. Fiber in the morning means less hunger late in the afternoon when you're most likely to overeat. This will also help you to stay mentally focused and maintain energy later in the day, keep your metabolism revving, and maintain steady blood sugar.

Tip 14- Swap the Soda

There are a lot of bad food and beverages being marketed these days, but soda is one of the worst. Did you know that one can of coke has more than 10 teaspoons of sugar? That is almost <u>double the recommended daily</u> total for an adult!! All of this added sugar can lead to diabetes, obesity, tooth decay, heart disease, hormone imbalances and many other health issues. This also includes diet soda which is equally as harmful so don't be fooled.

Instead of soda, try these alternatives: seltzer water with lemon wedge, unsweetened iced tea, or infused water with frozen fruit. These should satisfy your cravings without the added sugar and other artificial ingredients that soda contains.

Tip 15- Replace "bad" carbs with "good" Carbohydrates

All carbohydrates are NOT the same. There are two types of carbohydrates, simple and complex. You must eliminate poor (simple) carbs - those high in sugar & fat that quickly elevate insulin levels in the body. Examples of these would be white bread, pizza crust, pastries etc. Complex carbs are considered good in that they breakdown much slower in the body keeping insulin levels from spiking. Examples of these would be whole grains, fresh organic vegetables, fruits and legumes such as beans, peas, and lentils. Starchy, high sugar foods should be avoided not just for weight loss but for optimal health.

Tip 16- Buddy Up

Some of us have a difficult time staying motivated and on track when it comes to exercise. Having a friend, spouse, brother or sister, roommate or anyone else to partner with can be very valuable to your success. However, never forget that you always have to be most accountable to YOURSELF, as ultimately you are the one that has to decide to make changes to your health.

No one is responsible or to blame for de-railing your fitness routine except you. Have a pre-set time each day that you will work out together and be accountable for each other. Partner workouts are fun, make you train harder, and motivate you to want to continue. Don't forget to include some outdoor workouts to give you and your partner variety and prevent boredom.

Tip 17- Ditch the Scale

Too many people get obsessed with weigh-ins. You need to keep in mind that your weight can and most likely will sometimes fluctuate quite a bit (sometimes as much as 5-6 pounds) throughout a day. When you start a new fitness routine, it takes some time to see significant changes in the number on the scale. Also, when beginning a strength training program it is normal to have your weight increase slightly in the first few weeks as water increases to aid in helping inflammation and muscle repair. What's important is to consider all components of measuring fitness- body fat percentage, circumference measurements, and LBW (Lean Body Weight) or muscle.

Equally as important are those things that you can't measure such as having more energy, sleeping better, more self-esteem, better skin tone, and increase in libido. I recommend performing weigh-ins weekly or bi-monthly just to get a feel for progress and to be sure you are moving in the right direction.

When you stay consistent with exercise and eat nutritious foods, the weight will go down as a result so BE PATIENT.

Tip 18- Be Prepared

Being prepared is a step that can save you a lot of time and frustration. By planning your meals and snacks on the weekend for the upcoming week, blocking out your workouts on your calendar, and compiling a list of important tasks to complete are all things that will make for a more organized, less stressful and structured week.
These small things add up to big things and ultimately get you closer to your goals.

Finally, simple things like keeping a bag of healthy snacks and water in your car for when you are stuck in traffic or can't find a healthy lunch option can really come in handy and prevent the regret and extra calories of drive-thru food.

Tip 19- Follow the "80/20" Rule

It is pretty close to impossible to be super strict and eat clean all the time. I also don't recommend that you do it. It is important to balance your eating habits so that approximately 80% of the time you are eating nutritious foods that will fuel your body and give it the nutrients it needs and keep insulin levels steady. The other 20% you can deviate from this and not be so strict and splurge a little. I call this the "80/20 Rule".

This deviation will satisfy your cravings and prevent having to rely on willpower-which we already know doesn't work. This way you still give your body the necessary nutrients to perform at its best. Keep in mind you may have to experiment with the 80/20 rule to find what works best for your lifestyle and activity level.

Tip 20- See the Doctor

Do you get regular yearly checkups with your physician? Self- care is a very important habit to keep your body functioning like a well-greased machine! I recommend you have blood pressure, triglycerides, cholesterol, and thyroid levels tested at a minimum yearly. Know these numbers as it is important to track over time. Consult with your doctor if something doesn't feel right and always listen to your body, it speaks to you often so don't ignore it!

If you are working hard trying to lose weight and you don't seem to be making progress like you should, you may have an underlying medical condition. Take that short trip to your physician, it could be the solution that is hindering your efforts.

Tip 21- Recover

Allowing your mind and body to rest (recover) is a very important component to your health and wellness. Did you know that muscle building takes place when you are resting and not in the gym? It is during this time that your body repairs itself making you stronger, increasing muscle size, and replenishing glycogen-your body's fuel.

Recovery must occur before progress can be made. It's important for staying injury-free, long-term consistent training, and maxing out your weights from time to time.

The amount of time you need for recovery depends on several factors including exercise intensity, load, and frequency. Focus on your nutrition on your rest days and be sure you are drinking plenty of water to reduce soreness and inflammation.

Tip 22- Limit Stress

Stress is your body's way of responding to any type of demand or threat. This can be a good thing as when your body goes into "fight or flight" mode which is what protects us in a tense situation. However, most of the stress we carry has a negative impact on our body. Symptoms of this type of stress include weight gain, digestive issues, sleep problems, depression, mood swings and more.

There are several ways to manage stress which include daily exercise or physical activity, relaxation techniques such as meditation or yoga, eating a healthy diet, and getting enough quality sleep. All of these will help to control hormones and keep stress under control. Keeping a balance of work and leisure is also a good way to maintain a balanced lifestyle and limit stress.

Tip 23- Gut Check Time!

The importance of a healthy gut is a topic that hasn't been researched until just a few years ago. Your gut consists of millions of bacteria, both good and bad. The key is to keep these two balanced. Too much of the bad bacteria will cause inflammation in the body, digestion issues, and hormone imbalances. Millions of people suffer from an imbalance due to poor food choices.

Taking a quality probiotic supplement and reducing foods known to cause inflammation such as alcohol, fried foods, soda and other carbonated beverages, caffeine, and refined processed foods such as donuts and pastries will aid in reducing these issues.

Foods are a very important component to reducing inflammation in the stomach. Some of the best to include are foods rich in antioxidants such as blueberries, tomatoes, peppers, and tomatoes. Foods rich in vitamin B and calcium such as green leafy vegetables, and Greek yogurt are also good options.

Tip 24- Stretch Daily

Many of us have chronically tight muscles, primarily from sitting too much. This shortens and tightens muscles, decreases blood flow, and can cause other physical limitations. As we age, our muscles tighten and we lose range of motion.

Some of the benefits of stretching are:
1. Increases joint mobility and flexibility
2. Prevents common injury and pain management
3. Enhanced muscle function and performance
4. Improved circulation
5. Improved posture
6. Relaxation and stress relief

I recommend stretching every day. If this is difficult, try for 4-5 times per week. A regular stretching routine will keep muscles lengthened and make daily activities more enjoyable and reduce pain.

Tip 25- Color Up

We all know that we should be eating more fruits and vegetables. There are some vegetables that have a higher nutritional content consisting of fiber, vitamins & minerals and antioxidants that could be responsible for helping you live longer, feel and look better and prevent some diseases. These fruits have a darker color and are referred to as "super fruits". These include blueberries, acai berries, grapefruit, apples, tomatoes, cherries, and cranberries, just to name a few. Great choices for vegetables are broccoli, beets, kale, spinach, red peppers, and peas.

The best part is that most of these are readily available at your local market. I recommend buying organic whenever possible. Organic produce is grown without the use of pesticides, synthetic fertilizer, GMO's and other harsh chemicals used to preserve flavor and quality.

Tip 26- Be Consistent and Persistent

I can't tell you how important this one is. Consistency and persistence are how you succeed not just in fitness, but in life. Things never get easier, you just get stronger, find better ways to deal with obstacles and never give up. Growing stronger happens one day at a time, one small step at a time so be patient and when things don't go the way you would like just keep pushing, stay focused and don't give up!

One good habit to adopt is to go to bed and awake around the same time each day. Secondly, plan your next day's tasks the prior day or evening and try to complete important tasks earlier in the day when you are fresh and at your peak.

Tip 27- Start Small

From my experience, I see a lot of people fail at accomplishing a task or goal because they try to go too hard, too fast, or do too little planning.

For example, if weight loss is your goal start by changing one habit such as making sure you eat breakfast every day. Trying to re-design your whole exercise and/or nutrition plan in a few days or even a week you will most likely set you up for failure.

Start with small changes and over time they will have a very big impact on your health leaving you feeling more confident, healthier, and determined to conquer that next goal!

Tip 28- Brown Bag It

Preparing meals and taking them to work and on the road can save you hundreds of calories per day and several inches on your waist. Restaurants are in the business to make money, bottom-line. Although some places have adopted lower calorie options titled "lighter fare", most other items are loaded with Trans fats, artificial additives, and heavily processed meats. These are things you don't want to be putting in your body. Beware, "Lighter" does not always mean healthier.

If you have to hit the drive thru occasionally, be smart and remember this: Drive thru's put healthier less-profitable items on the bottom of the menu since we almost always read top to bottom. We typically feel rushed and usually order from the top of menu. Finally, avoid the "meal deals" and "super-size" deal options as these will usually double your calorie intake.

Tip 29- Learn Time Management

We all have 24 hours in our day and time is our most important asset. Don't waste it! Avoid what I call "time suckers"- things that consume your time that don't get you closer to your goals or accomplished daily tasks. Things such as watching television or browsing Facebook for several hours are examples. Try to limit the amount of time you spend doing these things by setting a timer and when it goes off, move on to more important things.

Other ways to manage time effectively include:
1. Create a daily plan the night before. This gives you a good overview of how your day will pan out.
2. Use a calendar and organizer. This helps you be on top of everything going on in your life.
3. Learn to say NO! Don't take on more than you can handle.
4. Set reminders for important tasks 10 minutes before they start.
5. Prioritize. You most likely can't do it all so put the more important tasks at the top.

Tip 30- Use an Activity Tracker

Activity trackers like the Fitbit and Samsung Fit2 are a great way to give yourself accountability and motivation to move more. These devices track your daily steps, approximate calories burned, heart rate, stairs, sleep habits, and more. The trackers also give you the ability to join an online community by participating in challenges, contests, discussion groups, and other benefits that give you motivation and your training a "fun factor".

There are several types on the market nowadays so do your homework and pick the one that is the best fit for your needs and lifestyle.

Tip 31- Get Outside Your Comfort Zone

We must be motivated to making lifestyle changes in order to get the true results we desire. In order to do this, we have to sometimes be willing to break out of our normal routines and push our bodies to do things that are "uncomfortable". It is then that growth and extraordinary things can happen. Remember this quote:

"A ship in a harbor is safe, but that is not what ships are for." Unknown

Be brave and try something you have never done before. It is normal to feel scared and hesitant. It is in these situations that we truly discover what we are capable of if we are willing to just try.

Tip 32- Forget Willpower

Science has proven that when we rely on willpower and deprivation, weight loss fails. You may occasionally shun away from that chocolate glazed donut but you can't expect every occurrence will have that outcome. Keeping a balanced nutrition plan following the 80/20 rule (Tip #19) will set you up for success.

Recent studies show that willpower is a myth. Scientists believe that when it comes to weight loss, it is positive behaviors that will help you shed those unwanted pounds. These include changing your daily habits, keeping a food journal, and having a positive attitude to stay motivated and on track.

Tip 33- Plan Weekly Menus

Most of us are very busy and lead hectic lives. Planning your meals at the beginning of the week saves you time and frustration after a long day. Planning ahead ensures that you have everything you need so you are not frantically throwing a meal together. It also gives you a chance to try different recipes and give more variety to your nutrition plan.

Tip 34- Believe in Yourself
"Believe you can and you're halfway there."
Theodore Roosevelt

One of my favorite quotes that is so true. You can prepare, stay dedicated and work incredibly hard, but if you don't believe in yourself this becomes a major roadblock in accomplishing goals. Your beliefs drive your behavior. If you think negative thoughts, whether from fear of failing, rejection, or embarrassment then you will not allow yourself to do what it takes to succeed.

Getting into the right mindset is a crucial step in your journey to a better body and life. As the saying goes.....where your mind goes...all else will follow.

Tip 35- Avoid Fad Diets

Diet is a four letter word! Most people start a diet program hoping to lose weight, so they slash calorie intake. In this process, our body actually works AGAINST us- increasing hunger and slowing metabolism, the opposite of what you want.

The biggest problem with these types of weight loss diets is that it is impossible to sustain and you always go back to where you were or sometimes worse. The "weight" that you lost in this short period was most likely water, not fat! So all that willpower and deprivation wasn't really worth it after all.

Finally, some diets will actually tell you not to exercise because the calories you are taking in are so few that you would not have the energy and it could be dangerous. Does that sound right? NO WAY. If you are looking to lose a few pounds rather quickly for an upcoming event or something, you can do this safely and successfully eating real whole foods in the proper portions.

Changing body composition requires some time and discipline in terms of eating healthy and exercise, but it is the only long-term way to maintain a healthy body weight consisting of lean muscle and body fat in the healthy range.

Tip 36- Minimize Processed Foods

Processed foods are stripped of valuable nutrients in the manufacturing process. Some foods are more heavily processed. Things such as white bread, packaged crackers, deli meat and pre-made frozen dinners would fall under this category. Other "processed" foods that are lightly processed due to convenience would be frozen fruit, bagged vegetables, or canned nuts. These can be acceptable options due to simplicity and higher shelf life.

Obviously, it would be best to avoid heavily processed foods and choose fresh fish, lean meats, fresh vegetables and other foods offered in raw state. These will give your body the necessary nutrients for sustained energy, improved digestion, and a better quality of life.

Tip 37- Reward Yourself

You have been diligent with your workouts, eating healthy and sticking to your routine, so reward yourself!   Hard work and discipline deserves to be rewarded so don't feel guilty. Go out and buy a new workout outfit or dress, plan a night out, buy a new surfboard, or whatever makes you feel good! The positive state of mind it creates will motivate you to keep going.

Tip 38- Limit Alcohol Use

Alcoholic beverages may hit the spot after a long day, however if weight loss is your goal alcohol (beer, wine and spirits) will definitely slow down your weight loss. Alcohol interferes with the fat-reducing process in the body and adds unnecessary calories to your diet, mostly through added sugars.

Although there are some health benefits to red wine, most people have a hard time sticking to one glass. If you do consume alcohol, try to limit it to only 2 or 3 glasses per week of wine or beer. You could also try some naturally flavored carbonated water with a lime or lemon wedge as this may satisfy your craving without the negative effects.

Tip 39-Think Habits, Not Diets

As I mentioned in tip 35, diets rarely are successful because they are short-term fixes. Actually, statistics show that 95% of diets fail. It is impossible to eat that way long term because your body is not designed to do this. You have to think long-term habits, not quick fixes for a healthy body and mind EVERY day of the year.

Adopting healthy daily habits will take discipline and some planning. Habits also take some time to develop so don't get frustrated and give up too soon. It used to be stated that it takes a minimum of 21 days to form a new habit. However, new research shows that it actually takes 66 days. Be persistent and patient and you will be happy that you stuck with it by being more successful physically and mentally.

Tip 40- Measure Progress

Progress is not strictly measured by the scale. There are so many other ways to measure success. At the beginning of your health and wellness journey be sure to record before photos, circumference measurements of the waist, chest, thighs, neck, & hips. When you are losing weight, the scale may not be going down as much as you would like, however you could still be making steady progress replacing stubborn fat with muscle.

Other ways of measuring progress is simply how your clothes are fitting, having more energy throughout the day, getting better quality sleep, and simply looking and feeling healthier! Keep all of these positive outcomes in mind rather than just focusing on the number on the scale.

Tip 41- Set a Routine

There is a lot of truth in the quote, *"Small daily improvements are the key to staggering long-term results"*. The routine that you perform daily is the most important tool you have to achieve your goals, whether short or long-term.

The specific daily habits you adopt and complete will compound over time and propel you forward to achieve success in your life. Daily habits provide structure and organization in your life giving you direction and meaning to create personal success.

Finally, routines prevent you from relying on motivation and willpower to get things done. Willpower is finite and motivation is not constant. Once you set up your routine, it is on autopilot and the need to practice willpower is not necessary.

Tip 42- Spend Some "Alone Time"

Setting some time aside by <u>yourself</u> can be very valuable. This includes turning off all electronics and cell phones as these will just distract your mind. Use this time to relax and relieve stress by doing some light stretching, yoga, listening to music, meditation etc. As little as 20 minutes per day will ease your mind and relieve stress leading to better health and productivity. Remember, too much stress leads to elevated cortisol levels, hypertension, sleeping disorders and other negative side-effects on your body.

Meditating can have such a profound effect on the body and mind. By seeking daily quiet time, you can recover faster from workouts, sleep better, feel less anxious and stressed, and have an overall better relationship with yourself and others. Why do it for "weight" loss? Meditation increases self-awareness so you're less likely to succumb to emotional eating when you're practicing meditation consistently.

Studies have shown that cortisol (the "stress" hormone) decreases during Transcendental Meditation, whereas it did not change significantly in control subjects during ordinary relaxation. When the stress hormones are high from prolonged habitual stress (which most of us are accustomed to), our bodies burn very little fat. When stressed, we reach for quick energy from sugars, caffeine and other simple carbohydrates in order to satisfy. A better option would be to close your eyes and do 20 minutes of relaxation meditation. It "recharges the batteries" and makes you feel great.

Tip 43- Avoid "fat free" Foods

In the last 10-15 years there have been a huge amount of products sold as "low-fat" or "fat-free". The problem with this is when fat is excluded it is replaced with sugar and other artificial ingredients to make it taste better. These ingredients can be detrimental to your health if consumed in large quantities. Ever since the inception of fat-free products, obesity and diabetes rates have steadily increased. Doesn't that tell you something?

"Fat-free" eating is not the answer to losing weight or staying lean. Eating real foods in the proper amounts is your best method.

Tip 44- Plan Pre and Post Workout Meals

What you eat before and after you exercise will have a big impact on results. Avoid large meals pre-workout as it will take your body longer to digest and you shouldn't exercise with a full stomach. Choose a small snack approximately 60 minutes before your workout. Good choices would be a piece of fruit, slice of toast with peanut butter, or a homemade granola bar. This is especially important if you are doing an early morning workout. At this time, your body has been in a fasting state for 8-9 hours so it's a good idea to have something small to jump-start the metabolism and give you some energy to make it through your workout.

Equally important would be your post-workout recovery meal. This can be in the form of a shake or food. Examples of some post-workout choices would be a protein shake made with a high-quality protein powder, a banana with tbsp. peanut butter, 8 ounces of chocolate milk with a piece of fruit, or turkey sandwich on whole wheat bread or tortilla.

The post-exercise goal is to replenish your glycogen (energy) stores and provide nutrients to muscles for growth and repair while you are in the recovery stage.

Tip 45- Limit Fried Foods

I think this one is pretty obvious, fried foods at fast food places are not on the clean-eating menu! Almost all will contain high amounts of saturated and trans-fats which can lead to heart disease, obesity, atherosclerosis and many other preventable diseases. Be sure to limit these types of foods in your diet. Choose the option of baked or grilled as these are a much healthier choice and less likely to add inches to your waistline and negatively impact your health.

Tip 46- Don't Be a Victim of "Excusitis"

We all have fallen into "excusitis" from time to time…making excuses for just about anything that becomes challenging or uncomfortable. Isn't it easy to just talk yourself out of doing these things? Will this get you closer to your goals or accomplishments? NO! Humans are creatures of habit and most people have daily habits that they rarely deviate from. When situations arise that knock us off this routine, we sometimes defend ourselves with excuses.

For example, don't ever use the weather as an excuse to miss a workout. Your health HAS to be a priority. Rain, hail, sleet, wind or whatever is just another excuse. Remember, you must stick to a consistent routine to reach your goals. It is your responsibility to act on them and make them become reality.

Tip 47- Learn From Failures

"I've missed more than 9,000 shots in my career. I've lost almost 300 games. 26 times, I've been trusted to take the game winning shot and missed. I've failed over and over and over again in my life. And that is why I succeed."
Michael Jordan

I love this quote from one of the best to ever play the game. Failing at something is never easy; however, there is a lot to be learned and you should embrace failure. Picture being successful in everything you have ever done in your life....would you be where you are today? Probably not. Learning from mistakes and failures is one of the best ways to overcome obstacles, grow stronger mentally and gain confidence. Some of the most famous people in the world have faced many failures. These adversities were used as lessons and helped them to grow into powerful, inspirational figures.

Next time you experience a failure, ask yourself this: What can I learn from this and how will I adapt and do differently so that I succeed the next time? Record these experiences in your journal for future reference.

Tip 48- Set Goals

Not setting goals is like jumping in your car without a destination! In order to know where you are going you must be prepared and make a plan. This is not specific to fitness or weight loss but for all other situations. Goals should be SMART (Specific, Measurable, Attainable, Realistic, Time-bound). Simply saying that you want to lose some weight is too generic. A better goal setting statement would be "I will lose 10 pounds by exercising 5 days a week and eating healthy for six weeks".

Successful goal setting involves two more important things:
1. Be prepared to perform a "goal audit" and re-evaluate your goals on a regular basis.
2. Reward yourself once you achieve a goal. (Treat yourself to a massage, new workout outfit, dinner at an upscale restaurant etc.). This will motivate you to keep going, especially when obstacles are thrown at you.

Tip 49- Use Apps

Nowadays, there are hundreds of great apps to help you stay organized, track calories, get nutritional information and lots more. Take advantage of these apps as they can help tremendously, especially with health and fitness. Most people have NO idea how many calories they consume throughout the day. Using apps to track your food such as MyFitnessPal, Fitbit, Lose it or Tap and track will give you a daily breakdown of what you are consuming. Enter your food from a database of thousands of items and it will record calories, fats, carbs, sodium & protein. At the end of the day/week you get a summary of all the valuable information.

Try it for a couple of weeks and you will be better informed and probably surprised at what you notice!

Tip 50- Create Healthier Versions

Nowadays there are hundreds of websites, blogs, and other resources related to nutrition and recipes. Adopting healthy eating habits does not always mean that you have to give up everything you enjoy! There are lots of recipes of healthier versions of your favorite foods out there so do some research. Simple substitutions can save you hundreds of calories and other un-healthy ingredients you don't need.

Here are a few of my favorite sites for healthy recipes:
www.mywholefoodlife.com
www.allrecipes.com
www.100daysofrealfood.com
www.skinnytaste.com

Be sure to bookmark these sites and print off your favorite dishes. By trying a variety of different foods from different food groups, you will have a well-balanced, nutrient-dense eating plan.

Tip 51- Eat Frequently, Not Enormously

The physiology of it has been known for years - when we starve ourselves, we get fatter. You probably have heard this before but it is worth repeating. Small meals throughout the day is the best way to keep your metabolism revving, give your body the nutrients it needs, burn fat, keep hormone levels constant, and prevent over-indulgences. When you skip meals and go 5 or 6 hours without eating your body will go into "starvation mode"- preserving calories and fat. This will shut down your metabolism and cannibalize hard-earned muscle- NOT what you want! In addition, because you have waited so long you are more likely to eat unhealthy foods and in large quantities.

Try to avoid going more than three hours without eating some small nutritious snack. Some healthy, easy snacks include raw nuts, fresh fruit, yogurt, protein bars, cottage cheese, or celery with peanut butter. As always, be sure to read nutrition labels to make sure you are staying within your limits.

Tip 52- Shop the Perimeter

Have you ever noticed that the freshest and greenest foods are on the outside "perimeter" of the market? This is where you should be buying the majority of your food items. Here you will find fresh fish and poultry, fruits and vegetables, lean meats, dairy and yogurts, and healthy deli items. These are the foods that should fill most of your shopping cart. Why? These types of foods have a higher nutritional content than the "ready to eat" foods found in the center isles. This helps you better control sugar, sodium and fat in your diet.

Finally, don't be mis-led by marketing labels and advertisements and always read food labels. Less ingredients, the better.

Tip 53- Skip the Gym

Although some may disagree with this one, you do not need to go to a gym to get great fitness results. Home workout programs are becoming very popular nowadays and are a great option to reach your goals. Working out at home saves you time, is convenient, gives you the ability to spend more time with family and saves money on a gym membership. With minimal equipment, you can achieve results, and have more time for important tasks and stay disciplined with your nutrition being closer to the kitchen.

Bodyweight workouts give you the ability to create a workout anywhere, anytime with minimal space. In addition, you are able to work multiple muscle groups at once, maximizing your calorie expenditure.

As a Beachbody coach, I help people from all over the country achieve their health and wellness goals with home-based fitness programs and nutritional supplements that deliver results.

Get Outdoors! Exercising outdoors is fun, boosts your mood, and has been proven to burn more calories. Go to your local park and you will see that there are a lot of opportunities to be creative with your training.

Tip 54- Eat More Fiber

Consuming more fiber will help you in many ways. Fiber acts as a "sweep" for your digestion track helping prevent irregularity and inflammation. Fiber also is important in weight loss and management as it helps you feel "fuller" by slowing carbohydrate metabolism preventing overeating and stabilizing blood sugars.

Research has also shown that including more fibrous foods in your diet lowers risk of developing kidney stones, heart disease, stroke and other diseases. The FDA recommends that adults consume at least 20-30 grams of fiber per day. However, recent studies have shown that 30-40g is more beneficial. Good sources include fresh fruits and vegetables such as leafy greens, avocados, peas, squash, nuts and seeds, beans and legumes. Be sure to drink plenty of water as well to flush your body and keep everything moving.

Tip 55- Don't Focus on Cardio Only

Cardiorespiratory exercise is very important and should be part of your routine. It strengthens your most important muscle- the heart. It also can reduce blood pressure, lower cholesterol, and increase your endurance- how long you can perform an activity.

However, you must add weight training to build lean muscle. It is difficult to build muscle from solely doing cardiovascular exercise. I outlined benefits of strength training in Tip #5 so go back and read again to see why weight training is a must for both men and women.

Tip 56- Start Your Day with Exercise

Kick-starting your day with exercise is a great habit to get into due to the many positive effects of exercise including boosting endorphins-your feel good hormone, sustained energy, and jump-starting your metabolism. You will also feel relieved and a sense of accomplishment by completing your workout earlier in the day.

When you put off your workouts until later in the day or evening, it can be too easy to find other "things" to do or just become too tired after a long day of work. If your schedule doesn't allow for a morning workout, late afternoon or early evening is the next best option.

Tip 57- Support Systems

Support systems are people that support, motivate, and encourage you with your health and wellness goals. This could be a workout partner, spouse, close friend, co-worker or anyone who keeps you accountable. This can be a very valuable tool when you encounter obstacles and setbacks, which you inevitably will.

Realize that it is normal to lack motivation and energy at times so having ways to cope with this is another way to stay consistent and on track.

Tip 58- Drink Green Tea

Green tea contains a plant compound called epigallocatechin-3-gallate (or EGCG) which promotes fat burning in the body. One study showed that people that had three to five cups a day for 12 weeks decreased their body weight by 4.6 percent or a loss of 2.2kgs without changing anything else. Other studies have showed benefits such as the prevention of certain cancers and diseases, increased cognitive function of the brain, and preventing heart disease and stroke.

For an extra antioxidant boost, squeeze in half a lemon's juice. Add a touch of honey for some sweetness as this could be a good way to satisfy cravings and control your weight.

Tip 59- Change Your Mindset

When it comes time to start a new exercise or nutrition routine you may encounter fear, confusion, or even frustration. Your body may be ready but your mind might be trying to talk you out of it! If this is true, you will need to work on the mental component in order to achieve long-term success.

Here are some things that may help motivate you and keep you on track:
1. Write down your weekly, monthly, yearly goals clearly.
2. Ask yourself…What is my motivation for making these changes? Record these in your journal.
3. Discuss your fears or roadblocks with your support systems. You don't have to do it alone. Seek out others that have gone through similar changes and ask for advice.
4. Remember your "why" for doing this. Record in your journal and post visual messages throughout your home or office.

Your mindset will determine your behaviors. Having all the knowledge in the world won't bring you life-changing results until you have the mindset to carry you through to success.

Tip 60- Take ACTION!

Sure, it's important to have beliefs, intent and desires but nothing happens until you take action. Let me repeat….NOTHING HAPPENS OR CHANGES UNTIL YOU TAKE ACTION! You are in charge of your life, no one else. Don't make excuses or blame others for not achieving success. Make today the day you vow to yourself that you will get healthy by exercising daily, reducing stress, and making nutrition a priority so that you can enjoy life without limitations.

Everyone has 24 hours in a day to do with it as he or she pleases. Don't waste time as time is the most valuable thing we have been given. Like a muscle, your motivation and discipline can be strengthened by your daily habits but not without ACTION.

I hope you enjoyed this book and found it valuable. Feel free to email me your thoughts, comments, or questions. I wish you all the best on your mission to better health.

DREAM BIG AND TAKE ACTION TODAY!

Pete Lyons

ACTION WORKSHEET

Using the tips you just read, complete the worksheet below to start putting these tips into practice. Remember, you can't make all these changes at once so start slowly with just a few at a time. Once you have implemented and established a new habit, move on to another one. Always remember these four words....YOU CAN DO THIS.

First 30 Days:

Goal 1:

I will get there by: _____

Goal 2:

I will get there by: _____

Goal 3:

I will get there by: _____

Goal 4:

I will get there by: _____

Goal 5:

I will get there by: _____